Artificial Intelligence In Drug Discovery And Development

Mbuso Mabuza

Published by Lekwandza Media, 2023.

ARTIFICIAL INTELLIGENCE IN DRUG DISCOVERY AND DEVELOPMENT

First edition. May 31, 2023.

ISBN: 979-8223379478

Written by Mbuso Mabuza.

Also by Mbuso Mabuza

A Healthy Mind And Best You: Achieving Great Results in Every Aspect of Your Life
Purposeful And Better You
Efficacy, Effectiveness And Efficiency In The Management Of Health Systems
Promoting Health and Wellbeing
Medicine and the Sociology of Health
Qualitative Methods In Public Health Research
Global Health Disaster Management
Global Health Policy And Programme Challenges
The Journey of Life Has a Gift of Purpose
Epidemiological Research
Ethics, Qualitative And Quantitative Methods In Public Health Research
Emotional Intelligence in Relationships
Blockchain Technology In Healthcare And Medicine
Immersive Technologies In Healthcare: Virtual Reality And Augmented Reality
Health Data Analytics And Informatics
How To Improve The Way You Think
Health Systems Engineering
Artificial Intelligence In Drug Discovery And Development
How To Make The Most Of Life
Precision Medicine
Connected Health: Technology-Enabled Care

Person Centered Care And Optimal Wellbeing
Reimagine Your Tomorrow
Leading Remote Teams in the 21st Century
Qualitative Research In Health and Medicine
Excellence In Medicine

Table of Contents

To the patients and families awaiting the breakthroughs of tomorrow. This work is dedicated to the visionaries striving to make faster, safer, and more accessible cures a global reality.

Where the limits of human cognition are reached, the horizon of artificial intelligence begins. In the dance between the silicon chip and the human cell, we find the blueprint for a new era of healing.

Preface

Artificial intelligence (AI) is a simulation of the process of human intelligence through computers.

AI has cemented its status as a powerful technology with the ability to propel a paradigm shift in healthcare and medicine of the 21st century and the future. The insights and values gained from AI and its subset, machine learning, are essential for predicting health outcomes and improving decision-making in healthcare and medicine.

AI can offer revolutionary insights into medicine, through data from genetics, proteomics and other life sciences that advance the process of drug discovery and development. Discovering drugs is a crucial first step in the biopharmaceutical value chain.

Drug discovery is a long, expensive and often unsuccessful process. The biopharmaceutical industry makes efforts to employ AI to improve drug discovery, reduce research and development costs, reduce the time and cost of early drug discovery, and support predicting potential risks/side effects in late clinical trials that can be useful in avoiding traumatic events in clinical trials.

The rapid growth in life sciences and machine learning algorithms has led to enormous statistical access to the growth of AI-based start-ups focused on drug innovation in recent years. The growing need to curb drug discovery costs and reduce time involved in the drug development process, the rising adoption of cloud-based applications and services, and the impending patent expiry of blockbuster drugs are some of the key factors driving the growth of this market.

However, shortage of AI workforce and ambiguous regulatory guidelines for medical software and lack of data sets in this field are some of the factors expected to restrain the growth of this market in the coming years.

Letter from the author

Dear Readers, Bloggers, Podcasters, Youtubers and Book Reviewers

Reading is a great way to personal growth, inspiration and healing. I was touched by a story of a man who read books during his mourning period following the death of his wife and children due to a car accident. I was also touched by a story of a woman who also read books during her chemotherapy treatment because it helped her to take her mind off her unpleasant procedure. Through her unwavering faith, she firmly believed that "life is a gift" in spite of what she had been through. Because of this, I put a sample of the book *'The Journey of Life Has a Gift of Purpose'* at the back of this book.

My hope is that my journey in writing will find my books in the hands of readers all over the world and touch hearts for the better.

Life has showed me that there is so much more to writing. The wonderful thing is that I have discovered a world of wonderful people with either a love of reading, writing, or both, so willing to share their opinions and be a catalyst to my writing.

Reviews are a tremendous influence online, and it would really help me reach my writing goal if you would please write a quick review of this book through your chosen online bookstore or platform. Your feedback tells me what you want to see more or less of. I believe we never stop learning. It is a lifelong gift to grow and change.

I want to invite you to join the mailing list to stay informed of all the new upcoming promotions and book give-aways.

Sincerely,

Mbuso Mabuza

mbusoprecio@gmail.com

Chapter 1
Overview of Artificial Intelligence

1.1 Introduction

While the phrase "artificial intelligence" has become a 21st century technological buzz-term, it was first coined by scientists at a conference in Dartmouth, United States of America, in 1956 during a conference which was arranged to bring luminaries in the fields of cybernetics, mathematics, formal reasoning and other related fields of academia together to explore problem-solving (Crighton, 2021).

Artificial Intelligence (AI) is a term used to describe a machine's ability to simulate human intelligence. It is a science and set of computational technologies that are inspired by – but typically operate quite differently from – the ways people use their nervous systems and bodies to sense, learn, reason, and take action. While the rate of progress in AI has been patchy and unpredictable, there have been significant advances since the field's inception over sixty years ago. Once a mostly academic area of study, twenty-first century AI enables a constellation of mainstream technologies that are having a substantial impact on everyday lives (Stanford University, 2016).

It is necessary to understand exactly how artificial intelligence and machine learning are individually defined. Machine learning is defined as the scientific discipline that focuses on how computers learn from data. Machine learning can be either supervised learning, which focuses on classification (e.g. sorting pictures into those with cats in and those with dogs in from a large set of images), and unsupervised learning. Unsupervised machine learning has no set outputs. The machine seeks to find patterns or groupings within unsorted data. Artificial intelligence is the broader umbrella under which machine learning lies, and which encompasses the use of technology to perform tasks that would usually require human intervention including sensing, learning, reasoning, and taking action (Bremmer, Gibbs and Mitchell, 2019).

The cumulative effects of Moore's Law mean that we now have computational power in the palm of our hand which dwarfs that used to put mankind on the moon. This immense ability to perform billions of calculations a second allows the use of decades' old mathematical tools to perform unique and highly accurate pattern recognition and analysis. In health data, this is allowing the ability to reveal associations and anomalies from previously thought random health data sets. Furthermore, the ability to create artificial neural networks (ANNs) and allow them to learn by trial and error, billions of times, creates software that evolves to solve complex problems in a nature akin to a child learning (Bremmer, Gibbs and Mitchell, 2019).

Artificial neural networks (ANNs) are the foundation of autonomous artificial intelligence. Their conceptualisation derives schematically from the functioning of the brain and neurons, in particular the encoding phase by the neural engrams, i.e. the capacity of a neural network to create memory according to the Hebbian principles. ANNs are computer algorithms that introduce numerical and statistical learning methods that themselves work through perceived stimuli and make decisions.

The simplest neural network is the perceptron. A typical neural network has an input layer, a hidden layer, and an output layer each composed of several neurons; this can go up to several thousands of neurons in each layer and up to several tenths of layer for the deepest structures. Each neuron has an input and an output, the output is a mathematical function of the input called the activation function. And each output is linked to the next neuron (input) by a connection which is weighted via a formula including a weight and a bias. The weights and biases are changed via training by back-propagation algorithm which retro-propagates the error calculated on the last layer between the expected answer and the one given by the ANN. The importance of connections between neurons increases or decreases over the training and the dataset used.

For example, the neurons in the input layer could represent the health information collected during the outpatients' clinics. The hidden layer represents the pathologies that deteriorate a specific function in an individual. And the output layer can represent the outcome of such a cluster of symptoms (on the risk for the life of the patient).

In the literature and since the last decades, we find different methods using ANN such as multi-layered perceptrons, sigmoidal multi-layer neurons, convolutional neural networks, Kohonen networks, Hopfield networks, etc.

Artificial intelligence and machine learning have excellent performance in tasks involving image interpretation, suggesting that medical specialties such as dermatology and radiology are one of the most promising applications of the technologies (Bremmer, Gibbs and Mitchell, 2019).

Patient monitoring is another application for artificial intelligence. Oxehealth, Oxford, UK, have created a medical device in Europe intended to perform spot observations of pulse and respiratory rate 'contact free' via optical and infrared sensors with no staff involvement. Its novelty means no published academic papers are available, but an unaudited case study of its use on an acute psychiatric ward showed improved in speed of observation collection and in the patient experience as they did not have to be woken to have their observations taken (Bremmer, Gibbs and Mitchell, 2019).

Some of the traditional sub-areas of AI are (Stanford University, 2016):

- Search and Planning: deal with reasoning about goal-directed behaviour Search plays a key role, for example in chess-playing programmes, in deciding which move (behaviour) will ultimately lead to a win (goal).

- Knowledge Representation and Reasoning: involves processing information (typically when in large amounts) into a structured form that can be queried more reliably and efficiently.
- Machine Learning: is a paradigm that enables systems to automatically improve their performance at a task by observing relevant data.
- Multi-Agent Systems: considers the question of how more intelligent systems interact with each other.
- Robotics: investigates fundamental aspects of sensing and acting – especially their integration – that enable a robot to behave effectively.
- Machine perception: has always played a central role in AI, partly in developing robotics, but also as a completely independent area of study.
- Social Network Analysis: investigates the effect of neighbourhood relations in influencing the behaviour of individuals and communities.
- Crowdsourcing: is yet another innovative problem-solving technique, which relies on harnessing human intelligence (typically from thousands of humans) to solve hard computational problems

The element of AI which has driven the field into the public consciousness is "deep learning". As the name suggests, deep learning networks are capable of learning, unsupervised, from data that is unstructured or unlabelled. The proviso is that they still first need to be "trained" in massive amounts of labelled data, which gives them the basis from which they can mathematically isolate and analyse patterns within subsequent huge sets of data – effectively "learning". The data input can be anything digital, from an image to a credit card purchase. The output is a response to a query – asking the machine to recognise a face in the image or verify the credit card purchase. This is the subset of AI which is helping develop technology like self-driving cars, for one, and assisting big companies to sift through mountains of data to gain insights about their customers or industries, help develop new products or deliver improved efficiencies (Crighton, 2021).

Although the separation of AI into sub-fields has enabled deep technical progress along several different fronts, synthesising intelligence at any reasonable scale invariably requires many different ideas to be integrated (Stanford University, 2016).

Artificial intelligence (AI) is unleashing the next wave of digital disruption. Global investment in AI skyrocketed to somewhere between $20 billion and $30 billion in 2016, with 90 percent of this spent on research and development and deployment, and 10 percent on AI acquisitions (Gadzala, 2018).

Gartner research suggests that AI and machine learning will eventually infiltrate just about every existing technology and analysts at the Industrial Development Corporation (IDC) predict that global investment in new intelligence technologies will exceed us$265 billion by 2023. The IDC also predicts that AI will be a key component of 90 percent of business software applications, and more than 50 percent of user interface interactions will incorporate some form of computer vision, speech recognition, natural language processing and augmented reality (Crighton, 2021).

It is projected that AI in healthcare will grow at an annualised 48 percent between 2017 and 2023. Artificial intelligence (AI) has cemented its status as a powerful technology with the ability to propel a paradigm shift in healthcare and medicine of the 21st century and the future. The insights and values gained from AI and its subset, machine learning, are essential for predicting health outcomes and improving decision-making in healthcare and medicine. Advances in Artificial

Intelligence and Machine Learning Technologies are likely to influence the way healthcare and medicine are delivered, in the sense that artificial intelligence will determine who delivers healthcare or medicine, and where and when healthcare and medicine are delivered. Ultimately, this points towards a shift away from the clinic and allows patients to access healthcare and medicine where they want, when they want it, and how they want it.

Integrating AI into the healthcare ecosystem allows for a multitude of benefits, including automating tasks and analysing big patient data sets to deliver better healthcare faster, and at a lower cost. As such, artificial intelligence presents boundless capabilities in healthcare and medicine, such as assisting clinicians to make accurate diagnostics faster and efficiently, the processing of large volumes of healthcare data or medical records much faster and efficiently in the context of healthcare service delivery, and prediction of future therapeutic drugs that could work efficiently (Phaneuf, 2021).

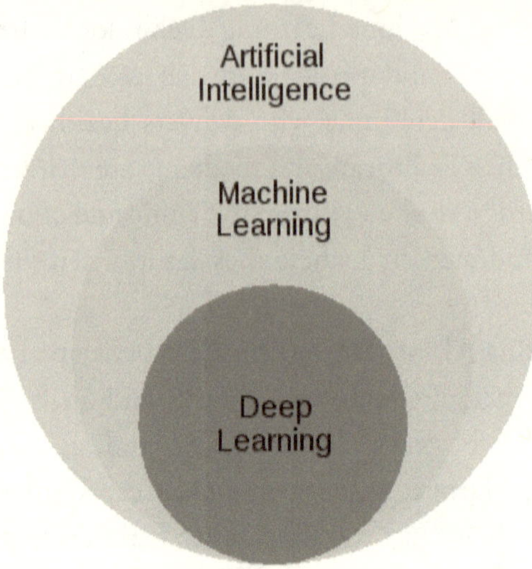

Figure 1.1 Artificial intelligence and artificial intelligence subfields as pieces put together

AI IS BEING USED OR trialled for a range of healthcare and research purposes, including detection of disease, management of chronic conditions, delivery of health services, and drug discovery. AI has the potential to help address important health challenges but might be limited by the quality of available health data, and by the inability of AI to display some human characteristics (Nuffield Council on Bioethics, 2018).

The use of AI raises ethical issues, including: the potential for AI to make erroneous decisions; the question of who is responsible when AI is used to support decision-making; difficulties in validating the outputs of AI systems; inherent biases in the data used to train AI systems; ensuring the protection of potentially sensitive data; securing public trust in the development and use of AI technologies; effects on people's sense of dignity and social isolation in care situations; effects on the roles and skill-requirements of healthcare professionals; and the potential for AI to be used for malicious purposes. A key challenge will be ensuring that

AI is developed and used in a way that is transparent and compatible with the public interest, whilst stimulating and driving innovation in the sector (Nuffield Council on Bioethics, 2018).

Like the web, artificial intelligence can be a positive force for political change, social change, and economic change. However, we need to ensure that all groups will also benefit from this technology. The problem today is that much of the discourse around artificial intelligence and its implications is taking place in North America and Europe (Thakur, 2018).

One tool that has been touted as a potential solution to meeting the expectations of growth or the demographic boom that is largely young and urban on the African continent is Artificial Intelligence (AI). As with many disruptive technologies, however, AI can be used for positive or negative ends. Delivering the promise of positive AI will require good systems of governance (Besaw and Filitz, 2019).

Artificial intelligence (AI) is changing society as profoundly as the steam engine and electricity have done. But unlike past technological revolutions, the AI revolution offers a unique chance to improve lives without opening up and exacerbating global inequalities. That will reduce widening of the locations where AI is done. The vast majority of experts are in North America, Europe and Asia. Africa, in particular, is barely represented. Such lack of diversity can entrench unintended algorithmic biases and build discrimination into AI products. And that is not the only gap: fewer African AI researchers and engineers means fewer opportunities to use AI to improve the lives of Africans. The research community is also missing out on talented individuals simply because they have not received the right education (Cisse, 2018).

Development and deployment of artificial intelligence in Africa is hampered by lack of connectivity, lagging technologically and other issues, but a handful of countries in the region such as Mauritius, South Africa, Seychelles, Rwanda and Senegal – spurred by the demand for economic development and recently by the need to combat COVID-19

- are laying the groundwork for innovation in the technology - making artificial intelligence a priority (Wright, 2020).

Perceptions of Africa as lagging technologically have been highlighted once again, this time by the release of the 2020 Government AI Readiness Index published by UK-based Oxford Insights. Only Mauritius, South Africa, Seychelles, Rwanda and Senegal make it into the ranking, and the report paints a gloomy picture of Africa "playing catch up in the area of artificial intelligence due to poor technological development, lack of infrastructure and a labour force that is not critical and innovative (Shearer, Stirling, Pasquarelli et al., 2020; Wright, 2020).

Africa faces several known challenges in developing AI such as a dearth of investment, paucity of specialised talent, and a lack of access to the latest global research. These hurdles are being whittled down, albeit slowly, thanks to African ingenuity and to investments by multinational companies such as IBM Research, Google, Microsoft, and Amazon, which have all opened AI labs in Africa. Innovative forms of trans-continental collaboration such as Deep Learning Indaba, which is fostering a community of AI researchers in Africa, Zindi, a platform that challenges African data scientists to solve the continent's toughest challenges, are gaining ground, buoyed by the recent "homecoming" of several globally-trained African experts in AI (Candelon, Bedraoui and Maher, 2021).

Yet, the central challenge that Africa faces in deploying AI is often overlooked: Africa's biggest companies – its national champions – are not zealously championing the cause of AI or deploying AI applications widely, causing them to trail behind global rivals. The few that have invested in AI have incurred above-average costs because they have imported talent and technology. Moreover, these companies are using AI only in limited ways. With limited bargaining power vis-à-vis foreign digital giants, and having failed so far to develop local talent, African companies run the risk of being less competitive than their multinational rivals in their home markets (Candelon, Bedraoui and Maher, 2021).

Today's company-specific AI gap will be tomorrow's national competitiveness chasm. Unless African companies actively drive the development of AI, African nations will never be able to leapfrog global rivals. Other nations have benefited from developing country-specific initiatives. Canada, Israel, and Singapore, for instance, have become globally competitive in AI by creating linkages between government, business, and academia. So can Africa (Candelon, Bedraoui and Maher, 2021).

Gender equity is critical to achieving AI fairness. Technological innovations such as artificial intelligence promise to identify and close the gender inequity gap through claims of a more data-driven, objective approach, but ironically pose another hurdle for women. Often, these digital systems inadvertently carry the same old analog gender biases (ICT Works, 2021).

There are now famous instances of the unintentional consequences of AI, such as automated resume screeners rejecting women, facial recognition disproportionately failing for women, and algorithmic credit-scores ranking women lower than men (ICT Works, 2021).

As AI tools are being tested and used in developing economies to drive insights and gain efficiencies across sectors – and as we rely more and more on them to give loans, diagnose diseases, triage medical care, and respond to humanitarian crises – we must work to prevent them from discriminating. There is an opportunity and urgency to optimise for innovative and equitable AI – especially in developing countries (ICT Works, 2021).

Development actors are taking steps to address disparities, for example, using AI to close gender-related data gaps in child marriage. Through the WomenConnect Challenge, USAID is beginning to tackle algorithmic gender bias in lending and is committed to taking action on the fair development and use of AI more broadly, working with partners to create a report and online course to better integrate AI fairness in development (ICT Works, 2021).

But we know there are many more ways that bias manifests in AI. Complex contributors to these harmful outcomes can include unrepresentative datasets, largely male data science teams, cultural norms around gender, and local policies and practices around data, among many others (ICT Works, 2021).

Responsible AI strives to be inclusive, rights-based, and sustainable in its development and implementation, ensuring that AI applications are leveraged for public benefit. Responsible AI will influence the future of information and communication technology for development.

Hearteningly for humans, Gartner's research indicates that AI and machine learning won't completely replace people because AI-driven autonomous capabilities cannot match the human brain's breadth of intelligence and dynamic general-purpose learning. Instead, they focus on well-scoped purposes, particularly for automating routine human activities (Crighton, 2021).

1.2 Expert Systems

Expert systems represent the lowest level of AI. Expert systems are comprised of a knowledge; an inference engine, which uses IF-THEN-ELSE rules to make sense of the dataset; and a user interface, where a user receives the required information. Such systems are best applied to automatic calculations and logical processes where rules and outcomes are relatively clear. 'Expert systems work the way an ideal medical student would: they take general principles about medicine and apply them to new patients" (Obermeyer and Emanuel, 2016). Despite relatively simple technology behind, expert systems could be very powerful in medical assistance. Many patient-oriented medical chatbots are based on expert systems: Florence is a practical chatbot for older patients that reminds them to take their pills (Florence – your health assistant, 2018). SafedrugBot embodies a chat messaging service that offers assistant-like support to doctors who need appropriate information about the use of drugs during breastfeeding. Efficient diagnosis assistant systems are also based on expert systems: bots like

Your.Md or CitizenDoc aim to help patients find a solution to the most common symptoms through AI. However, a chatbot never replaces an experienced doctor. If the patient's issue seems severe or doubtful, the bot itself addresses the user to an appointment with a diagnosis and eventually for the prescription of a therapy. In a specific domain concerning millions of patients with sometimes difficult access to care, some authors have described an algorithm to screen tuberculosis, based on a rule base, knowledge base, and patient database architecture. All these expert systems are based on a relatively recent subfield of computer science called machine learning.

1.3 Machine Learning Algorithms and Paradigms

Machine learning, gives "computers the ability to learn without being explicitly programmes."

As a field of study, machine learning sits at the crossroads of computer science, statistics, and a variety of other disciplines concerned with automatic improvement over time and inference and decision-making under uncertainty (Jordan and Mitchell, 2015). The uncertainty of a diagnosis inferred from a sign could be basically seen as a mathematical problem dealing with probabilities. The application of probability theory to learning from data is called Bayesian learning (Ghahramani, 2015). An algorithm is trained to execute a task (e.g., to distinguish cancer from non-cancer tissues) and to improve its performance and accuracy with experience. Depending on the amount of data and computational live judgement. Machine learning techniques often deal with a large amount of data and therefore, have a more realistic approach of biological and medical problems than "simple" mathematical science and modelization.

Three different paradigms can be classically described in machine learning. These are supervised learning, unsupervised learning, and a combined method referred to as reinforcement learning.

1.3.1 Supervised Learning

In supervised learning, the algorithm focuses on a known output; in that case the goal is to produce a probabilistic prediction *y'* in response to a query *x'*. Supervised machine learning models are trained on a pre-labelled data referred to as the training set of (*x*, *y*) pairs. The training error is roughly defined by the difference between predicted outcome y' and actual outcome y. Supervised learning systems form their predictions via a learned mapping *f(x)*, which produces an output y for each input *x*. Supervised learning includes several probability algorithms, like decision trees, decision forests, logistic regression, support vector machines, neural networks, kernel machines, and Bayesian classifiers (Jordan and Mitchell, 2015). The classical example in medicine is the automated interpretation of an ECG or a CT scan. These are all tasks that a trained physician can do and so the computer is often trying to approximate human performance (Deo, 2015) *and maybe surpass it*. The number of parameters of such a model is critical: more parameters reduce bias but increase noise (and random associations). The complexity of a model is a trade-off between bias and variance (Jordan and Mitchell, 2015).

The medical applications of supervised learning are diagnosis assistance for rare, difficult pathologies, and also follow-up, that needs an accurate evaluation of treatment outcome: one application on children diagnosed with cerebral palsy with support vector machines shows an overall accuracy of 96.80% in diagnosis using only two easily obtainable basic gait parameters (Kamruzzaman and Begg, 2006). Similarly, the diagnosis of valvular heart disease through neural network ensembles has been made with an accuracy of 97.4% (Das et al, 2009).

1.3.2 Unsupervised Learning

In contrast, in unsupervised learning, there are no outputs to predict. The goal is to find patterns or groupings within the data. No training is needed because there is no desired output. The underlying concept is called clustering, that is to say, the assumptions that among a dataset, the machine can automatically regroup features (symptoms, images, genes). A criterion function is defined as one that embodies these assumptions

– often making use of general statistical principles such as maximum likelihood, the method of moments, or Bayesian integration – and optimisation or sampling algorithms are developed to optimise the criterion (Jordan and Mitchell, 2015).

The "fuzzy" aspect gives the algorithm the flexibility to classify a data point to each cluster to a certain degree relating to the likelihood of belonging to that cluster. This method can detect hidden patterns across large and complex datasets. Unsupervised learning can be very useful in identifying mechanisms or risk factors for complex multifactorial diseases (Deo, 2015). Fuzzy c-means (FCM), an effective clustering method developed by Bezdek (Turing, 2018), is one of the most common instruments for medical diagnosis (Wu et al, 2015). It has already been proposed for classification of thyroid diseases (Azar and El-Said, 2013) or tumours by gene characterisation (Sun and Xu, 2014). This method also has its weaknesses: the need to determine membership cut-off, i.e., the distance from the feature to the centre of the clusters, roughly represented by the mean of the considered data and the fact that clusters are formed whatever the inputs, i.e., if the data belong to no cluster at all, the algorithm will do it anyway, thus potentially leading to errors. FCM has shown its efficiency in primary headache, where diagnosis is often difficult. The algorithm showed an accuracy (proportion of true results – whether positive or negative) of 0.97 for migraine (Wu et al, 2015).

1.3.3 A Combined Method: Reinforcement Learning

Instead of training examples that indicate the correct output for a given input, the training data in reinforcement learning are assumed to provide only an indication as to whether an action is correct or not. The action taken by the algorithm is reinforced by a reward if it is correct; if the action is incorrect, the problem of finding the correct one remains.

1.4 DEEP LEARNING

Unsupervised learning and reinforcement learning are the fundamental principles for deep learning that are applied among successive layers of the dataset. Dee learning discovers intricate structure in large datasets by using the back-propagation algorithm to indicate how a machine should change its internal parameters that are used to compute the representation in each layer from the representation in the previous layer (LeCun et al, 2015). Deep learning can therefore offer an exciting solution to incomplete biomedical knowledge: these methods can discover new biomarkers without any human input, conceivably generating truly unexpected discoveries (Oakden-Rayner et al, 2017).

Some algorithm results have demonstrated similar performance to human experts in the assessment of diabetic retinopathy, dermatological lesions (Esteva et al, 2017), atrial fibrillation screening (Halcox et al, 2017), or Parkinson's disease (Ma et al, 2014).

1.5 ALGORITHMS FOR Decision-Making

Medical knowledge and publications are increasing exponentially. As explicitly describe by Mesko: "in 1950, it was estimated that the doubling time for medical knowledge was about 50 years. In 1980 it was about 7 years for medical knowledge to double. In 2010, it only took about 3.5 years. It was estimated that by the year 2020, it would take only 73 days for the volume of medical knowledge to double". In the domain of physician trained in epidemiology, it would take an estimated 627.5 hours per month to evaluate 23 million articles on PubMed (Alper et al, 2004). The quantity of medical knowledge is simply impossible for a person to retain even if this person was reading the material all day long, whereas a computer program can read all the data, store the relevant information, and use it to help in medical decision-making. These kinds of algorithms are based on the natural language processing (NLP); they can understand a text written by a person and extract intent, sentiment, or meaning.

The IBM AI program, Watson, launched its special algorithm for oncologists able to provide clinicians evidence-based treatment options. The purpose is to support tumour board meetings: "Watson for Oncology has an advanced ability to analyse the meaning and context of structured and unstructured data in clinical notes and reports that may be critical to selecting a treatment pathway, combining attributes from the patient's file with clinical expertise, external research, and literature data" (Mesko, 2017).

1.6 Algorithms in Radiology: The Era of Radiomics

Traditionally, medical imaging has been a subjective or qualitative science. Nowadays, the amount of imaging datasets combined to computational methods provides a comprehensive quantification combined to visual assessment (Larue et al, 2017). The use of computational algorithms to analyse medical images is now called "radiomics" (Oakden-Rayner et al, 2017; Kumar et al, 2012; Lambin et al, 2012). Even if the authors may not all agree with the extent of this new domain, a large definition of radiomics can include two machine learning-applied procedures: classical image analysis with human eyes-defined features which is derived from supervised learning and deep learning with feature learning, whose principle is close to an unsupervised learning (Oakden-Rayner et al, 2017).

Response evaluation criteria in solid tumours (RECIST) is a set of published rules that define cancer evolution during treatments, and was originally published in February 2000. Nowadays, the many clinical trials evaluating cancer treatments for objective response in solid tumours are using the RECIST platform, which is developed by Parexel Informatics. This kind of standardised criteria, still dependent on the physician's observation, can be considered as the first step to replace the radiologist's eye by the computer. In magnetic resonance imaging (MRI), some research in prostate cancer has shown that textural features were significantly correlated with Gleason score (Gnep et al, 2017; Wibmer et al, 2015).

In supervised radiomics, the methodology can be resumed in four steps: image acquisition, extracting radiomics features from the images, training the computer and validating a prognosis score. The extracting stage still needs human experts' intervention as image features still are human-defined features.

These "image features" are mathematical descriptions of the visual properties of an image, describing the low-level visual information present in an image, such as the intensity / brightness and the texture of image regions (Kumar et al, 2012; Lambin et al, 2012).

A radiomic biomarker definition requires robust approaches that analyse all of the available variations in an image. Deep learning appears to be an ideal tool to accomplish this goal.

Chapter 2

Drug and Vaccine Discovery and Development

Drug discovery is the first step of the value chain that identifies new candidate therapeutics for treating or curing human diseases. It is a long, expensive and often unsuccessful process. Drug discovery generally comprises four stages (research and discovery; clinical development; manufacturing and supply chain; launch and commercialisation; postmarket surveillance and patient support). Theses stages take five to six years to complete, excluding the initial drug target identification and assay development steps, which are largely driven by academic and other research centres. It is the initial stage of biopharma research and development and involves the identification and optimisation of potential new drugs and a preclinical *in vivo* validation through cell assays and animal models. Successful candidates that meet the regulatory requirements applied to drug discovery move into the clinical trial phase, where they are tested for efficacy and safety in humans (Deloitte, 2019).

Drug development is the process of bringing a new drug molecule into clinical practice; in its broadest definition, it includes all stages from the basic research of finding a suitable molecular target to large-scale Phase III clinical studies that support the commercial launch of the drug to post-market pharmacosurveillance and drug repurposing studies. During the drug development process, chemical entities that have the potential to become therapeutic agents will have to be identified and thoroughly tested, and the entire process is lengthy and costly. It is estimated that for every new drug brought to the market, it typically costs billions of US Dollars and more than 10 years of work. As such, drug discovery is a long, expensive and complex process with a very low success rate. Therefore, strategies that can facilitate and accelerate the drug development process are of high interest (Chen et al, 2017).

People who are very ill often need the newest medicines or therapeutic drugs in the healthcare pipeline. As such, bringing new medicine to patients struggling with serious illness is the driving force behind medicines or therapeutic drugs discovery and development. However, developing new medicines or therapeutic drugs and shepherding them through the regulatory process is expensive. What is more, it can take several years, usually between ten to fifteen years to bring a new medicine or therapeutic drug to market. For this reason, there is tremendous interest when it comes to finding ways to develop medicine or therapeutic drugs with higher throughput methods. These days, though, computer simulations can speed up the development and regulatory evaluation of pharmaceuticals and medicinal products. This can make the process more efficient for medicines' developers and manufacturers. This eventually helps patients, as well, especially those who desperately need newly developed medicine or therapeutic drugs to treat their patients.

Recent advances in the field of AI have fuelled the emergence of new methods to accelerate the drug discovery process. The vast chemical space that is available to sample drug-like molecules can be efficiently explored using a combination of AI-based methods (Bung et al, 2021).

Vaccines are biological preparations that confer immunity against specific diseases, typically by provoking a response from the body's immune system. The immunogenic vector can be an attenuated or dead form of the pathogenic microorganism, parts of microbes, or microbial deoxyribonucleic acid (DNA), or compounds that mimic microbial products. Exposure to such pathogens induces the production of immune cells with pathogen specificity that the body retains for long periods of time. These immune cells provide for a rapid response upon subsequent exposure. In other words, vaccines lead to the development of immune memory, by simulating the threat of an infection and thus providing antigens derived from the specific pathogen (WHO, 2016).

Vaccines against non-communicable diseases – an emerging field of research and development – also work by modulating the human immune system. These target cells, proteins, or other molecules, rather than pathogens or pathogen-infected cells (Stevens et al, 2017).

Vaccination has been in use for centuries. In the 16th century, Chinese physicians treated healthy people with ground smallpox scabs to reduce their chances of infection during epidemics. In 1796, the English physician Edward Jenner, who successfully inoculated an eight-year-old boy with exudate from a cowpox lesion, succeeded in providing the principle scientifically (Stevens et al, 2017).

Vaccination is a powerful method of disease prevention that is relevant to people of all ages and in all countries, as the COVID-19 illustrates. Vaccination can improve people's chances of survival, protect communities from new and re-emerging health threats, and enhance societal productivity. But achieving the promise of vaccination requires much more than the vaccines themselves. It requires appropriate incentives to encourage the timely discovery and development of innovative, effective, safe, and affordable products; effective financing and delivery programmes; and credible scientific leaders who can provide evidence-based policy recommendations and reassure the public about the value of the vaccines (Gerberding and Haynes, 2021).

Because vaccines are usually administered to healthy people, maintaining the highest safety standards is not only an ethical imperative but is also essential to sustaining public trust. The story of vaccine progress has been punctuated by both real and misguided safety concerns for as long as vaccines have been in use. Such concerns have included adverse events associated with vaccination itself, quality lapses in the manufacturing process, and false alarms regarding vaccine safety. The potential for financial gain has fuelled liability suits related to putative safety concerns. Sustaining vaccine safety and trust will become increasingly complex. Vaccines continue to be approved, and more vaccines have become accessible in resource-limited countries, but safety surveillance systems are less evolved in many low-income regions than in high-income regions. Similarly, vaccines are being manufactured in regions where regulatory oversight is not always optimal, and counterfeit vaccines remain a threat. Emerging infections may require rapid availability of new vaccines before comprehensive safety studies are complete (Gerberding and Haynes, 2021).

The impact of innovations in medicines/drugs discovery and development on healthcare and society encompasses the following categories: clinical effectiveness; healthcare provider aspects, patient safety and security, economic and financial aspects; organisational aspects, socio-cultural aspects, legal and regulatory aspects.

Drugs developed using innovative (adaptive, patient-centric, precision medicine and real-world data) trials are more likely to be launched. Trial efficiency is improved by the adoption of innovative trials, although impact varied according to each innovation type and therapy area. Innovation has a foothold everywhere as innovative trials are being carried out across the globe, even though the European Union and the United States of America contribute the greatest proportions of trials within each innovation area. Innovation-using drugs are viewed favourably by payers and therefore, more likely to be adopted by payers. The findings indicate that the optimisation of innovations in drug discovery and development requires the ability to identify and balance nuances and trade-offs, rather than employing a "one-size-fits-all" strategy (The Economist Intelligence Unit, 2018).

While repurposing of existing drugs may be an option for developing new agents against neglected tropical diseases, widespread drug resistance is a major challenge in drug discovery and development, more so, for a repurposed drug (Weng, Chen and Wang, 2018).

"Amid the current situation whereby demand for antibiotics far outweighs supply, it is critical to spur global innovation of new antibiotics, alternative therapies and diagnostic tools in order to address the growing challenge of antimicrobial drug resistance (Renwick, Simpkin, and Mossialos, 2016).

While Europe and the United States of America have invested heavily in antibiotic research and development, it is still unclear how the heavy investment has impacted outcomes, and it is also unclear how Europe and the United States of America will share in future profits of such investments should their funding result in marketplace products. The antibiotic research and development environment is now crowded, and there is room for improvement regarding coherence and coordination between and within initiatives, as analysis shows that a far greater number of push incentives are used over pull incentives leading to an unequal distribution of initiatives across the antibiotic value chain (Renwick, Simpkin, and Mossialos, 2016).

There remains a need for even greater harmonisation between regulatory agencies. The findings suggest that antibiotic conservation and patient access objectives are poorly integrated into the existing innovation schemes recommendations are that (Renwick, Simpkin, and Mossialos, 2016):

- Existing and new antibiotic research and development initiatives should be aligned to function within the broader One Health approach to antimicrobial drug resistance (AMR).

- Existing and new European antimicrobial drug resistance initiatives and antibiotic research and development initiatives, including clinical trials should be consolidated under a One Health approach.

- A global antimicrobial drug resistance policy coordination and governing body that brings worldwide coherence under a One

World approach to antimicrobial drug resistance should be established.

- Efforts to coordinate and expand European and global antibiotic clinical trials programme under One Europe and One World agendas should be intensified; ensuring that antibiotic incentives are explicitly attached to specific high-priority medical needs in infectious diseases.

- Ensuring that antibiotic incentives reinforce global stewardship and access goals.

- Push and pull incentive mechanisms should be linked in a hybrid approach to stimulating antibiotic research and development.

- A global antimicrobial drug resistance and antibiotic pipeline data, shares knowledge and disseminates best practice in AMR and antibiotic innovation should be launched.

- European and global commitment to antibiotic pull incentives should be registered; the role of European joint procurement of high-value antibiotics should be explored to ensure their conservation.

- The feasibility of European tax policies that encourage antibiotic research and development should be considered; methods of clawing back public investment in antibiotic research and development should be incorporated into incentive packages.

- Cooperation and harmonisation across global drug regulatory agencies for licencing novel antibiotics should be improved.

- Key market weaknesses should be addressed by further enabling small and medium enterprise participation and facilitating preclinical development.

- The incentive preferences of different industry players should be explored.

- The value of different partnership models in antibiotic research and development should be investigated and there should be learnings from the experiences of the Biomedical Advanced Research and Development Authority, Innovative Medicines Initiative, Joint Programming Initiative on Antimicrobial Resistance" (Renwick, Simpkin, and Mossialos, 2016).

Efficiency of clinical trials can improve as technology tools improve communications not just with staff but with patients and communities. Other areas that could be impacted positively by technology in clinical trials include recruitment, retention, delivery of intervention, and data collection (Rosa et al, 2016).

The benefits show that mHealth will improve data quality in the trial, patient trial adherence, patient engagement, safety and signal detection. As mHealth or digital health technology availability increases in the healthcare arena, adoption rates and benefits remain unclear (Henderson, 2015).

This is affirmed by Oracle Health Sciences (2017) who highlight five main benefits of incorporating mHealth technology into clinical trials: real time data capture; improved data quality; real world evidence from continuous data; increased insight into patient adherence; reduced monitoring effort via remote monitoring

"One of the major challenges for the pharmaceutical industry, today, is the huge cost of research towards discovering and developing a new medicine or therapeutic drugs. The main reason for this challenge is that despite considerable advancement in technology, there are complexities facing that face drug discovery and development, and this also indicates that there is a glaring innovation deficit within the pharmaceutical industry, in that regard. The 'Core Model', an economic and organisational paradigm for drug discovery and development is elucidated through its three major elements: the 'core' (representing the company's internal resources and people who are hired because they have assets related to the core's objective of making drugs), the 'bridge' (representing the immediate collaborators of the core and the private institutions to which the core has indirect access through the external collaborators), and the 'periphery' (an open, public and cooperative system, containing the institutions or agencies interested in what the core has to offer for the benefit of society, as well as the funding and regulatory structures that support the core and the bridge).

An innovative network science that addresses the general need for improved applications in the discovery and development of drugs is proposed as the survival of the pharmaceutical industry and of the world's healthcare systems will ultimately depend on innovation, on a better understanding of disease, on the efficient development of novel drugs and on preventive measures coupled to an efficient use of the limited societal resources. While the utopian thought of imagining a world free of disease is nowhere near our distant sight, the question of whether it is achievable or not, still remains" (Sanchez-Serrano, Pfeifer and Chaguturu, 2018).

The high cost of research in the pharmaceutical industry remains a huge challenge as it is estimated that it takes on average, more than $2.558 billion and 10-15 years to develop a new medicine or therapeutic drug. Since the actual cost of specific drugs is not disclosed to the consumers, it is difficult for the consumer in the pharmaco-dependent society to know which drugs required more investment than others, as the consumer who accesses a new drug is almost always required to pay a premium (Sanchez-Serrano, Pfeifer and Chaguturu, 2018).

Sustained competition between start-ups and big pharmaceutical players is viewed by industry leaders as an unwelcome disruption as it potentially reduces the drug discovery and development share market of big pharmaceutical companies. In hindsight, the disruption is also viewed as an opportunity for big pharmaceutical companies to re-position themselves and come up with new business models as the start-ups collapse and fail to survive in a fast changing and more diverse environment. At the same time, another view is that even if the business model can survive, but not at the same scale as the large-scale limits innovation because it creates incentives to protect successes to pay off failures and not to innovate (Munos and Orloff, 2016).

Given the increasing cost of bringing a new drug to the market, and the declining and stagnant research and development productivity, there is urgent need for disruptive innovation by identifying and rapidly bringing new and affordable drug discoveries to the market. Some of the complex challenges facing the pharmaceutical industry such as the sustained competition from generic drug manufacturers and the overall negative public reactions to costly drugs only fuel the complexity of drug discovery and development (Munos and Orloff, 2016).

Qualitative research interviews with leaders from a range of positions in the drug development ecosystem yielded some insights on the complexity of the challenges facing drug discovery and development. While there was consensus about the significant challenges facing the drug discovery and development industry, there were varied views about the breadth and pace of transformation needed. Although there was growing optimism about the state of the pharmaceutical enterprise, there was apprehension about start-ups bringing their models and breaking into the market as such tends to disrupt the market shares of already established players.

The argument was that if it became cheaper to innovate new drugs, there will be more diversity but reduced scale as many players will enter the field, but few start-ups will survive, and the established players will eventually thrive amidst the disruption, and a complex ecosystem will emerge based on a revitalised business model. There will be a more patient-centric decentralised model that will enable patients to have a strong voice as they become more engaged, and such advances will transform drug discovery research encouraging non-hypothesis-driven research. In the context of healthcare delivery, it was envisaged that the pharmaceutical industry was better positioned to influence healthcare service delivery to be more efficient. The bottom line was that changing the cost structure was paramount to a transformed drug discovery and development enterprise (Munos and Orloff, 2016).

To curb the issue of high cost, lengthy processes and competition with start-ups, many big pharmaceutical companies have opted for repurposing existing drugs for other indications with the aim of developing new therapeutic agents against neglected tropical diseases (Weng, Chen and Wang, 2018). Other perspectives are that there is great benefit in employing successful strategies which involve the mechanism of 'Push' which aims at cutting the cost of research and development for industry and 'Pull' which aims at increasing market attractiveness (Weng, Chen and Wang, 2018).

"New digital technologies are transforming Alzheimer's disease clinical trials. Digital technologies have been shown to improve data quality and enhance guidance during the administration of a test by proactively responding to errors, calculating results automatically, managing branching rules, checking for consistency of responses, and responding immediately to missing data. They also enable the management of translations and the integration of audio and video data capture into assessments. The end result of using digital data capture is an increase in both accuracy and precision, both of which are necessary to detect anything other than large effect sizes. Digital technologies using gaming approaches can enhance screening to subtle cognitive changes. Patient engagement, recruitment and compliance can be improved through digital technologies. Digital biomarkers are already being used as secondary end points in clinical trials for neurological disorders. The other advantage of digital technologies in clinical trials is that it enables the deriving of insights from complex data (Gold et al, 2018).

"There are various benefits of e-technology in clinical trials. Efficiency of clinical trials can improve as technology tools improve communications not just with staff but with patients and communities. Other areas that could be impacted positively by technology in clinical trials include recruitment, retention, delivery of intervention, and data collection. Other important benefits of using e-technology in clinical trials include less cost per patient as the clinical trials are conducted faster, fostering research and development, effective and efficient platform for all stakeholders involved in the research enterprise, facilitation of implementation and dissemination as the technology helps expand both the recruitment of participants as well as the reach of scientific discoveries to those who may not otherwise have access to it (Rosa et al, 2016).

While there are areas of promise there are also limitations of digital clinical trials. There are privacy/confidentiality issues. Keeping up with technology may be a challenge as what was revolutionary when the clinical trial started may be utterly obsolete by the time it is finished, leaving results, even when positive, of limited applicability. Including a non-representative sample as using technology in research is that participants recruited from social media and online sites are not a representative sample for studies and that this may introduce bias. Adequate infrastructure may not be possible as we- or mobile-based interventions also require the use of different types of infrastructure and resource support, which can be difficult to navigate. Issues of big data and accuracy of data may be a limitation given the sheer quantity of data available, one of the biggest challenges is to identify which data to collect, how to capture it, and how to analyse it. User identification is one of the biggest complexities that come when users online have the ability to be mostly or completely anonymous can increase the comfort required for some to participate in unfettered dialogue, it can also make it difficult to verify identities or specified demographics in a study population. Provider attitudes can be a challenge as time limitations for researchers and stigma about professionalism can be barriers to the use of blogs and social media as well" (Rosa et al, 2016).

"There are five main benefits of incorporating mHealth technology into clinical trials that are highlighted: real time data capture; improved data quality; real world evidence from continuous data; increased insight into patient adherence; reduced monitoring effort via remote monitoring (Oracle Health Sciences, 2017).

The benefits show that mHealth will improve data quality in the trial, patient trial adherence, patient engagement, safety and signal detection. As mHealth or digital health technology availability increases in the healthcare arena, adoption rates and benefits remain unclear (Henderson, 2015).

Challenges include ethical concerns such as privacy and data sharing, informed consent, disclosure, conflicts of interest, and ownership of data. The regulatory path for digital technologies is unclear. There are many other challenges that need to be considered. There are no empirical data to show that digital devices could get answers more quickly in phase 2 studies; there is need for new tools to have novel metrics, not simply improvements to the older tests; obtaining normative data in older people is difficult because many older people have comorbid conditions; collecting and analysing massive amounts of data may be impractical; when collecting data from patients, timing is crucial because people have good days and bad days and different cycle times; gaining acceptance from physicians may interfere with workflow; and usability testing of digital devices and applications with representative sample of users may be a challenge" (Gold et al, 2018).

Challenges and barriers to mHealth adoption in clinical trials are large and complex, and they can be divided into business barriers and technical barriers. The business barriers include lack of regulatory clarity or acceptance; organisational resistance to change; increased cost or lack of return on investment; ability to make effective use of data collected; concern over ability for vendors to scale beyond pilots. The technical barriers include lack of FDA approved sensors and wearable; data security issues; lack of integration with EDC-CDMS; Scalability – collecting, storing, cleaning, submitting; lack of medical sensors for a therapeutic area" (Oracle Health Sciences, 2017).

Other important benefits of using e-technology in clinical trials include less cost per patient, as the clinical trials are conducted faster, fostering research and development, effective and efficient platform for all stakeholders involved in the research enterprise, facilitation of implementation and dissemination as the technology helps expand both the recruitment of participants as well as the reach of scientific discoveries to those who may not otherwise have access to it (Rosa et al, 2016).

Increased cost or lack of return on investment could be a threat for adopting digital clinical trials in healthcare and medicine (Oracle Health Sciences, 2017).

There are no empirical data to show that digital devices could get answers more quickly in phase 2 studies; there is need for new tools to have novel metrics, not simply improvements to the older tests; obtaining normative data in older people is difficult because many older people have comorbid conditions; collecting and analysing massive amounts of data may be impractical; when collecting data from patients, timing is crucial because people have good days and bad days and different cycle times; gaining acceptance from physicians may interfere with workflow; and usability testing of digital devices and applications with representative sample of users may be a challenge (Gold et al, 2018).

Low consumer confidence can affect the implementation of digital clinical trials in both developed and developing countries. The term "clinical trials" is increasingly viewed with disdain by many people in developing countries due to ethical concerns and the unsavoury history of regarding the developing world such as the African continent as a "testing laboratory". As such, there is growing resistance towards anything to do with clinical trials from the perspective of the African diaspora.

Provider attitudes can be a challenge as time limitations for researchers and stigma about professionalism can be barriers to the use of blogs and social media as well (Rosa et al, 2016).

There are privacy/confidentiality issues. Keeping up with technology may be a challenge as what was revolutionary when the clinical trial started may be utterly obsolete by the time it is finished, leaving results, even when positive, of limited applicability. While there are areas of promise there are also limitations of digital clinical trials. Including a non-representative sample as using technology in research is that participants recruited from social media and online sites are not a representative sample for studies and that this may introduce bias. Adequate infrastructure may not be possible as mobile-based interventions also require the use of different types of infrastructure and resource support, which can be difficult to navigate. Issues of big data and accuracy of data may be a limitation given the sheer quantity of data available, one of the biggest challenges is to identify which data to collect, how to capture it, and how to analyse it. User identification is one of the biggest complexities that come when users online have the ability to be mostly or completely anonymous can increase the comfort required for some to participate in unfettered dialogue, it can also make it difficult to verify identities or specified demographics in a study population (Rosa et al, 2016).

Lack of FDA approved sensors and wearable; data security issues; lack of integration with EDC-CDMS; Scalability – collecting, storing, cleaning, submitting; lack of medical sensors for a therapeutic area (Oracle Health Sciences, 2017).

Ethical concerns such as privacy and data sharing, informed consent, disclosure, conflicts of interest, and ownership of data (Gold et al, 2018).

Lack of regulatory clarity or acceptance is a growing issue of concern in both developing and developed countries (Oracle Health Sciences, 2017). There was an almost similar finding by Gold et al (2018) who observed that the regulatory path for digital technologies such as digital clinical trials was unclear. After careful analysis of planned regulations or regulations that are being implemented in certain countries and regions, it is worrying that there is ambiguous liability as there is no case law or no indication of who will be liable if things go wrong with digital clinical trials.

As such, there is need to focus on education and quality standards for both providers and consumers in the healthcare and medicine ecosystem. Even if there were to be globally applicable regulations for digital clinical trials, such regulations would fall short because it is not possible to rationalise as different countries or regions require different formulas.

Weng, Chen and Wang (2018) acknowledge that neglected tropical diseases are complex, and, yet, there is insufficient innovation for neglected tropical diseases. Notable highlights of the study are the importance of collaborative efforts in discovery; efficient approaches for drug innovation; policy advocacy; technology advancement in drug discovery; successful strategy for drug innovation; and novel financing models in drug discovery. The product development partnership model now plays a crucial role in drug innovation, which usually involves research institutions, pharmaceutical companies, government agencies and international organisations. Collaborative innovation via the open source mechanism is an indispensable way to coordinate various stakeholders towards a common target of discovering and developing new drugs to combat the spread of neglected tropical diseases.

The lack of transparency of the pharmaceutical industry in terms of sharing information and doing the right thing for patients remain challenges. In that regard, consumers have lack of trust in the drug discovery and development industry. The pharmaceutical industry is often viewed as serving a certain agenda to appease some of the big developed countries with big economies. Talks of piloting potential drugs in the developing world by big pharmaceutical companies headquartered in Europe or north America sparks controversies and conspiracies about the developing countries being treated as 'guinea pigs', used to experiment the efficacy of potential new medicine and drugs. For example, there was great unease among many Africans when the news of testing a potential vaccine against the COVID-19 started making the rounds. Some of the legends of African football made the views known in protest against big pharmaceutical companies such as the one based in France after confirming their intention to test a potential vaccine against COVID-19 in Africa. The question is, why is Africa used as a testing ground by big pharmaceutical companies based in the developed countries, and why is the testing not conducted in those developed countries?

Guidelines and government-regulated standards of normal expectations for different steps of the drug discovery and development process are in general readily available (Sanchez-Serrano, Pfeifer and Chaguturu, 2018).

In conclusion, judging from the staggering failure rate of experimental medicine or therapeutic drugs in clinical trials despite huge investments in novel technologies, productivity gains in the pharmaceutical industry remain elusive, indicating the stark reality that the pharmaceutical industry is facing a serious innovation deficit. As such, this points towards an urgent need for breakthrough innovations at the drug discovery and development front, in the battle against many of the diseases that inflict humanity (Sanchez-Serrano, Pfeifer and Chaguturu, 2018).

It is affirmed that the use of interactive multimedia has a significant effect in making study subjects understand information of clinical trials and participation. Although the effect of an improved understanding of the information was significant in general terms, it was more pronounced in children. This suggests that interactive multimedia may be a better way of engaging children in a manner that is familiar to them and which can enhance their ability to provide assent (Tait, Voepel-Lewis and Levine, 2015).

Chapter 3
Future Perspectives

While still in the early stages of adoption, artificial intelligence and machine learning technologies algorithms are showing promise in medicine.

Bringing new medicines or therapeutic drugs to patients suffering with rare or serious illness is the driving force behind new medicines or therapeutic drugs discovery and development. However, discovering and developing new medicines or therapeutic drugs is expensive and takes long before the successful new medicine or therapeutic drug comes to market. It is for that reason that high-throughput technologies in new medicines or therapeutic drugs discovery are a good prospect. Not surprisingly, cures for rare diseases are not often a priority for pharmaceutical companies when the return on investment is difficult to achieve for a small number of patients. In some cases, however, repurposing generic drugs as therapies for rare diseases can be a pragmatic and life-changing solution to this problem (Larkin, 2016). Much as there is no silver bullet innovation, the right innovations in drug discovery and development can and do have an impact on healthcare and medicine (The Economist Intelligence Unit, 2018).

Over the past few decades, tremendous effort has been put into developing agents to address the multidrug resistance mechanisms. The pharmaceutical industry is under pressure owing to the reduced output of new drugs, rising research and development costs, current economic recession, and stricter regulatory guidelines (Kamal et al, 2017).

Advances in artificial intelligence methods, especially in deep learning, have prompted studies that consider heterogeneous data sources and types such as clinical data, imaging, -omics data, and knowledge bases among others, in one coherent model. Technologies incorporating artificial intelligence have become versatile tools which can be applied universally in various stages of drug development, including identification and validation of drug targets, designing of new drugs, drug repurposing, aggregating and analysing biomedicine information and refining decision-making process to recruit patients for clinical trials, and prediction of feasible synthetic routes for drug-like molecules (Ahuja, 2019; Kamal et al, 2017).

The use of causal modelling tools in artificial intelligence, such as causal diagrams, could provide important additions to the implementations of causal inference using real-world data (RWD). Causal modelling can also lead to improvements in the interoperability and adaptability of artificial intelligence models in these drug development studies. This concept of causal artificial intelligence has been applied successfully in public health studies, such as the identification of occupational risk factors and the prediction of diarrhoea incidence in children among others, and could be potentially used in future drug development research such as the target trial framework aiming to establish causal treatment effects using real-world data without conducting randomised controlled trials (RCTs). Additionally, the emerging of explainable artificial intelligence (XAI) could help to interpret and understand artificial intelligence decisions. Explainable artificial intelligence models are particularly useful for tasks such as drug repurposing because these tasks are generating hypotheses where plausible explanations are crucial (Kamal et al, 2017).

Experts strongly believe that artificial intelligence will permanently change the pharmaceutical industry and the approach to discover new drugs. With artificial intelligence, the possibility of linking regenerative medicine with pharmacology and gene therapy emerges (Ahuja, 2019).

Some of the big pharmaceutical companies have now adopted an approach to research and development which focuses on the science related to the immune system, the use of human genetics and the application of advanced technologies, such as artificial intelligence and machine learning, to deliver transformational medicines and vaccines. This distinctive approach has enabled these pharmaceutical companies to strengthen their pipeline in vaccines and specialty medicines and accelerate the pace at which they discover, develop and deliver for patients (GSK, 2020).

Moving forward, vaccines against a range of infectious agents will need to be developed. New and emerging pathogens, such as SARS-Cov-2 and new influenza strains, regularly appear. Viruses that are capable of spreading by vector or airborne routes – one of the most important pandemic threats – continue to emerge (Gerberding and Haynes, 2021).

It is clear from the COVID-19 pandemic that nations need to be part of a rapid response system to discover and develop vaccines for novel threats and ensure they have a resilient supply of vaccines and antibodies for infectious threats new and old. For vaccines to play an effective part of pandemic recovery and preparedness, they must be available quickly, be manufacturable at scale, and be accessible to all people (Department for Business, Energy & Industrial Strategy, 2020).

Information technology (IT) offers the ability to treat and organise large amounts of data and leads to a paradigm of integration – in opposition to reduction – to explain biological systems and phenomenon (Andre, 2019). Quantitative datasets of DNA, RNA, proteins, and metabolites provide an unprecedented starting point to understand the effects of perturbations on a cell (Sauer et al, 2007) and, with addition of clinical tests and imaging, the effect on the whole body. The informational view of biology defines biological information – biomarker – as a given data integrated in a network. This leads to a "systems" approach to physiology and pathophysiology. It means changing our philosophy, in the full sense of the term (Noble, 1960).

Systems biology is then a holistic approach to deciphering the complexity of biological systems that starts from the understanding that the networks, which form the whole of living organisms, are more than the sum of their parts (so-called reductionism). It is collaborative, integrating many scientific disciplines – biology, computer science, engineering, bioinformatics, physics, and others – to predict how these systems change over time and under varying conditions (ISBUSA, 2018).

With the present emerging artificial intelligence (AI) technologies, computational "machine learning" techniques for training and generalisation from data, and cutting-edge statistical techniques, will play a significant role in analysing multidimensional datasets generated by the new technologies of systems medicine (Schadt et al, 2010). This progressively but rapidly leads to a "new taxonomy," generating new approaches for disease diagnosis, therapy, and clinical decisions, promising more individualised treatments and improved outcomes for patients (National Research Council Committee on AFfDaNToD, 2011). Indeed, if this approach becomes efficient in clinical practice, it provides a real paradigm change in health care, from reactive to proactive medicine. This proactive approach is already promising in "long-term" management of diseases: chronic illnesses (Sagner et al, 2017), infectious diseases (Bengoechea, 2012), or cancer (Tian, 2012).

The concept of "4P" medicine, that is predictive, preventive, personalised, and participatory, has been advocated since more than a decade now (Andre, 2019).

Actually, the 4P medicine concept has emerged from the convergence of three trends (Flores et al, 2013):

- The increasing ability of systems biology and systems medicine to decipher the biological complexity of disease: Each pathology is seen as a personal experience and a dynamic network which is dysregulated from health to disease, and

conversely, treatment is a pathway from disease to health, considering each personal dimension from molecular to social and its participation in the pathological state.
- The increasing ability of computers to integrate, store, analyse, and communicate data from medical records, symptoms, clinical tests, biological samples, imaging, and molecular biology: Then, a personalised data cloud can be imagined, including multiple dimensions of each individual, from genetic to phenotypic characteristics, but also sociometrics (social, education, familial context, etc.).
- The increasing access to information for patients and consequently their interest in managing their own health. The digital tools not only connect recent science fundamental discoveries to clinical applications but also the patients and health-care consumers. There is an increasing phenomenon for people to go online to investigate a medical condition (Fox and Duggan, 2013).

Drug research could also benefit from these tools. Indeed, the omics data analysis would not only allow the identification of new biomarkers representative of pathologies but also propose new therapeutic targets for the development of more effective drugs (Andre, 2019).

Precision Medicine, sometimes called personalised medicine, is an emerging technological advancement which aims to personalise prevention and treatment according to the genetic, environmental, and lifestyle variability of individual persons or a specific group of people with commonalities, as opposed to the one-glove-fits-all approach which has less consideration for the uniqueness of the individual person or specific group of people with commonalities such as similar genetic changes in a tumour. The genetic changes are determined in a special laboratory where a biopsy from the diseased organ or tissue is analysed through a process of DNA sequencing, genetic testing or molecular profiling. Once the genetic testing is completed, tailored treatment can be decided for the patient.

Perhaps, the clearest utility of precision medicine approaches thus far has emerged from efforts to improve disease diagnosis with the promise of better treatment. This perspective emerged as a critique of medical practices characterised as employing reductionist and oversimplified methods of disease categorisation (Ramaswami, Bayer and Galea, 2018).

Treatment is not the only aim of precision medicine, but prevention is also important as genetic testing for people with a family history of a certain illness such as diabetes mellitus, could also receive tailored preventive measures before those people even get sick. As such, precision or personalised medicine is driven not only by individual health data, but also by the availability of reference medical knowledge and evidence, that is, precision or personalised medicine is linking knowledge with individual health data for decision support (Kalda et al, 2015).

As such, precision medicine debunks the one-glove-fits all or clinical treatment paradigm which is a trial and error approach wherein all individuals presenting with some constellation of symptoms receive a similar treatment. Contrary to the precision medicine approach, the clinical treatment paradigm purports that a certain treatment should be given for a certain disease, such as antiretroviral therapy for people living with HIV, chemotherapy and radiation therapy for people suffering from cancer, and is oblivious of the unique genetic changes, environmental factors, lifestyle and behavioural factors of the individual and the adverse events that ensue.

Although personalised medicine has been there even during Hippocrates' time, where the emphasis was on giving the right medicine, to the right person, and at the right time; historically, the concept of modern day personalised medicine was first mentioned in a monograph title in 1998. While some of the field's core concepts date back to the early 1960s, the basic idea can be credited to the Canadian physician,

Sir William Osler (1849-1919) who recognised that no two individuals react or behave alike under the abnormal conditions we know as disease (Primorac et al, 2020).

The current evolution of personalised medicine is happening at a fast pace, whereby it goes beyond therapeutics selection for a patient but into the realm of drug discovery, planning and delivery of care, and engagement between consumers and companies focusing on the improvement of healthcare. Such rapid evolution of personalised medicine is largely driven by advances in diagnostics, digitalisation, data and analytics operating across a broad scope.

In recent times, the explosive growth of precision or personalised medicine has ceased to be just a basic science but it has incorporated -omics such as the correlations of protein expressions and specific diseases at cellular level (proteomics), how the molecular composition of certain genes are responsible for the production of certain proteins (genomics), and how certain metabolic processes at cellular level are associated with the expression of certain diseases (metabolomics). Ultimately, in precision medicine, the aim of understanding genomics, proteomics and metabolomics is to customise medical practice with a focus on the individual, based on the use of genetic tests, identification of biomarkers, and development of precisely targeted individualised drug treatments (Iriart, 2019).

Precision medicine then seeks to incorporate technology into medicine to create a data ecosystem that can better identify, treat, an individual patient's disease. This approach aims to seamlessly integrate clinical phenotypes and biological information, from imaging to laboratory tests (including –omics data) and health records. The rationale is to develop a new taxonomy of human disease based on molecular biology (Ramaswami, Bayer and Galea, 2018).

Over the past decade, precision medicine approaches have received significant investment to create new therapies, learn more about disease processes, and potentially prevent diseases before they arise. However, in many ways, precision medicine investments may come at the expense of existing public health measures that could have a greater impact on population health. As we tackle burgeoning public health concerns, such as obesity, and chronic diseases, such as cancer, and diabetes, among others, it is not clear whether precision medicine is aligned with public health or in conflict with its goals (Ramaswami, Bayer and Galea, 2018).

Nonetheless, precision or personalised medicine can be considered as the cornerstone of modern medicine. With so many hospital admissions being attributed to a 'one-size-fits-all' prescribing approach and adverse drug reactions being among the leading causes of death globally, not to mention the huge economic implications this creates, a tailored approach for every patient is needed. At the centre of this should be pharmacogenomics with the goal to improve drug safety and efficacy. Furthermore, therapy for each patient should be designed according to their personal characteristics, health status, lifestyle and pharmacogenetic profile. Ultimately, the goal of precision or personalised medicine is to contribute towards preventive, predictive and participatory health systems (Primorac et al, 2020; Kalda et al, 2015).

References

Ahuja, A.S. (2019) The impact of artificial intelligence in medicine on the future role of the physician. *PeerJ*, 7: e7702.

Ahuja, V. (2019) Artificial intelligence (AI) in drug discovery and medicine. *Journal of Clinical Cases and Reports*, 2(3), pp. 76-80.

Altshuler, J.S. & Altshuler, D. (2004) Organizational challenges in clinical genomic research. *Nature*, 429, 478-481.

Andre, A. (2019) *Digital medicine.* Springer

Azar, A.T et al. (2013) Fuzzy and hard clustering analysis for thyroid disease. *Comput Methods Prog Biomed*, 111(1), 1-16.

Besaw, C. & Filitz, J. (2019) *AI & global governance: AI in Africa is a double-edged sword.* United Nations University, Centre for Policy Research.

Big Data Value Association (2016) *Big data technologies in healthcare.* TF7 Healthcare subgroup, 21 December.

Bremmer, R., Gibbs, A. & Mitchell, A.R.J. (2019) The era of immersive health technology. *EMJ Innov*, 4(1), pp. 40-47.

Bung et al. (2021) De novo design of new chemical entities for SARS-CoV-2 using artificial intelligence. *Future Medicinal Chemistry*, 13(6), pp. 575-585.

Candelon, F., Bedraoui, H.E. & Maher, H. (2021) Developing an artificial intelligence for Africa strategy. Development Matters Africa. Available from: https://oecd-development-matters.org/2021/02/09/developing-an-artificial-intelligence-for-africa-strategy/

Chen, Z. et al. (2017) Applications of artificial intelligence in drug development using real-world data. *Drug Discovery Today*, PMID: 33358699.

CHT (2019) The ultimate guide: artificial intelligence in healthcare.

Cisse, M. (2018) Look to Africa to advance artificial intelligence. *Nature*, 562 (7728), p. 461.

Cornell University, INSEAD, and WPO (2019) *Global innovation index 2019: creating lives – the future of medical innovation*. Ithaca, Fontainebleau, and Geneva.

Cossy-Gantner, A., Germann. S., *et al.* (2018) Artificial intelligence (AI) and global health: how can AI contribute to health in resource-poor settings? *BMJ Glob Health*, 3:e000798. doi:10.1136/bmjgh-2018-000798.

Crighton, T. (2021) *AI: The real deal- artificial intelligence is starting to look less artificial.* Technically Speaking.

Daman, R., Tripathi, M.M. & Mishra, S.K. (2016) Cloud computing for medical applications & healthcare delivery: technology, application, security and swot analysis. *IJCSIT Conference Proceeding.*

Deloitte (2019) *Intelligent drug discovery: powered by AI.* Deloitte University EMEA CVBA.

Department for Business, Energy & Industrial Strategy (2020) *UK vaccine taskforce 2020 achievements and future strategy*. End of Year Report.

Deo, R.C. (2015) Machine learning in medicine. Circulation, 132, 1920-1930.

Dsouza, R. (2016) Evolution of robotics in medical surgeries and health care systems: a review. *International Journal of Applied Engineering Research*, 11 (23), 11277-11298.

Eccles, S. (2019) *Artificial intelligence in healthcare*. Academy of Royal Medical Colleges, July.

Economic Commission for Africa, African Union Commission, African Development Bank and United Nations Development Programme (2015) *Africa data consensus*. Addis Ababa: Economic Commission for Africa. Available from www.uneca.org/sites/default/files/PageAttachments/final_adc_-_english.pdf.

Eistevski, B. & Chen, M. (2018) Big data analytics in medicine and healthcare. Journal of *Integrative Bioinformatics*, 20170030.

El aboudi, N. & Benhlima, L. (2018) Big data management for healthcare systems: architecture, requirements, and implementation. Advances in Bioinformatics, https://doi.org/10.1155/2018/4059018

Esteva, A. et al. (2017) Dermatologist-level classification of skin cancer with deep neural networks. Nature, 542, 115-8.

Florence – your health assistant (2018) https://www.florence.chat

Fogel, A.L. & Kvedar, C. (2018) Artificial intelligence powers digital medicine. *npj Digital Medicine*, 1:5.

Gerberding, J.L. & Haynes, B.F. (2021) Half-century of progress in health: the National Academy of Medicine at 50. *New England Journal of Medicine*, 384, pp. 393-396.

Ghahramani, Z. (2015) Probabilistic machine learning and artificial intelligence. Nature, 521, 452-9.

Ginsburg, P.B. et al. (2018) The opportunities and challenges of data analytics in health care. *Brookings*, November.

Girard, M. (2019) *Big data analytics need standards to thrive: what standards are and why the matter.* Centre for International Governance Innovation. CIGP Papers 209, January.

Gnep, K. et al. (2017) Haralick textural features on T2-weighted MRI are associated with biochemical recurrence following radiotherapy for peripheral zone prostate cancer. J Magn Reson Imaging, 45(1), 103-17.

Gold, M. et al. (2018) Digital technologies as biomarkers, clinical outcomes assessment, and recruitment tools in Alzheimer's disease clinical trials. *Alzheimer & Dementia: Translational Research & Clinical Interventions*, 1, 234-242.

Gong, J. et al. (2020) A tool for early prediction of severe coronavirus disease 2019 (COVID-19): a multicentre study using the risk normogram in Wuhan and Guandong, China. *Clinical Infectious Diseases*, 71(15), pp. 833-840.

GSK (2020) *We are a science-led global healthcare company*. Annual report. GlaxoSmithKline plc.

Guo, J & Li, B. (2018) The application of medical artificial intelligence technology in rural areas of developing countries. *Health Equity*, 2.1: 174-181.

Halcox, J.P.J. et al. (2017) Assessment of remote heart rhythm sampling using the AliveCor heart monitor to screen for atrial fibrillation: the REHEARSE-AF study. Circulation, 136(19), 1784-94.

Henderson, L. (2015) The use of mhealth in clinical trials. *Applied Clinical Trials*, February/March Hoodbhoy, Z., Hasan, B. & Siddiqui, K. (2019) Does artificial intelligence have any role in healthcare in low resource settings? *Journal of Medical Artificial Intelligence*, 2:13.

ICT Works (2021) *Have you experienced gender inequity in artificial intelligence applications*? USAID.

Inan, O.T. (2020) Digitising clinical trials. *Digital Medicine*, 3:101.

Independent Expert Advisory Group on the Data Revolution for Sustainable Development (2014). *A world that counts: mobilising the data revolution for sustainable development*. Available from www.undatarevolution.org/wp-content/uploads/2014/11/A-World-That-Counts.pdf.

Indiana University (2019) *Biomedical analytics*. School of Informatics and Computing. https://soic.iupui.edu/courses/info-b585/

ISSA (2018) *Shaping the future of social security in the digital age*. 15th ISSA International Conference on Information and Communication Technology in Social Security, Casablanca, Morocco, 18-20 April.

Jain, D. & Singh, V. (2018) Feature selection and classification systems for chronic disease prediction: a review. *Egyptian Informatics Journal*, 19, 179-189.

Jiang, F., Jiang, Y., Zhi, H., *et al.* (2017) Artificial intelligence in healthcare: past, present and future. *Stroke and Vascular Neurology*;0: e000101. doi:10.1136/svn-2017-000101.

Jordan, M.I. & Mtchell, T.M. (2015) Machine learning: trends, perspectives, and prospects. Science, 349(6245), 255-60.

Kamal et al. (2017) *Future of drug discovery*. In: G. Aurora et al. (eds.), Drug Resistance in Bacteria, Fungi, Malaria, and Cancer. Springer.

Kamruzzaman, J. & Begg, R.K. (2006) Support vector machines and other pattern recognition approaches to the diagnosis of cerebral palsy gait. IEEE Trans Biomed Eng, 53(12 Pt 1), 2479-90.

Kappen, T.S. et al. (2018) Evaluating the impact of prediction models: lessons learned, challenges, and recommendations. *Diagnostic and Prognostic Research*, 2:11.

Kappen, T.H. et al. (2016) Barriers and facilitators perceived by physicians when using prediction models in practice. *Journal of Clinical Epidemiology*, 70, 136-145.

Kar, U. & Dash, R. (2018) Application of artificial intelligence in healthcare: past, present and future. *Archives in Biomedical Engineering & Biotechnology*, 1(1): 2018.ABEB.MS.ID.000503.

Kerr, R.S.C. (2020) Surgery in the 2020s: implications of advancing technology for patients and the workforce. *Future Healthcare Journal*, 7(1), pp. 46-49.

Kong, N. (2020) *Biomedical analytics and systems optimization research lab*. Purdue University.

Kumar, V. et al. (2012) Radiomics: the process and the challenges. Magn Reson Imaging, 30(9), 1234-48.

Lacombe, D. et al. (2017) Precision medicine: from "omics" to economics towards data-driven healthcare – time for European transformation. *Biomedicine Hub*, 2 (suppl 1), 480117.

Lai, M.C., Brian, M. & Mamzer, M.F. (2020) Perceptions of artificial intelligence in healthcare: findings from a qualitative survey study among actors in France. *Journal of Translational Medicine*, 18(14).

Lambin, P. et al. (2012) Radiomcs: extracting more information from medical images using advanced feature analysis. EUR J Cancer, 48(4), 441-6.

Larkin, M. (2016) *Repurposing drugs helps patients with rare diseases*. R&D for Pharma & Life Sciences. Elsevier.

LeCun, Y. et al. (2015) Deep learning. Nature, 521, 436-44.

Leung, M.K.K., et al. (2016) Machine learning in genomic medicine. *Proc IEEE*, 104, 176-197.

Liu et al. (2019) A comparison of deep learning performance against health-care professionals in detecting diseases from medical imaging: a systematic review and meta-analysis. *Lancet Digital Health*, 1: e271-97.

Luthra, H. et al. (2021) New paradigm in healthcare industry using big data analytics. *IOP Conference Series: Materials Science and Engineering*, 1099(2021) 012054.

Ma, C. et al. (2014) An efficient diagnosis system for Parkinson's disease using kernel-based extreme learning machine with subtractive clustering features weighting approach. Comput Math Methods Med, 2014:985789.

Mane, R.R. & Kulkami, R.V. (2012) A review: electronic medical records (EMR) system for clinical data storage at health centers. *International Journal of Computer Technology & Applications*, 3 (5), 1837-1842.

Martin, B. (2019) How to rid artificial intelligence of human prejudice. *OpenMind*, 13 November. BBVA.

McLellan, S. (2014) Precision medicine: the future of data-driven healthcare. Umea University.

Mesko, B. (2021) *Top 10 medical innovations of the future*. The Medical Futurist Institute Oberrmeyer, Z & Emanuel, E.J. (2016) Predicting the future – big data, machine learning, and clinical medicine. New England Journal of Medicine, 375, 1216.

Mesko, B., Hetenyi, G. & Gyoffy, Z. (2018) Will artificial intelligence solve the human resources crisis in healthcare? *BMC Health Services Research*, 18:545.

Mesko, B.A. (2017) A guide to artificial intelligence in healthcare. The Medical Futurist, Editor.

Munos, B.H. & Orloff, J.J. (2016) *Disruptive innovation and transformation of the drug discovery and development enterprise.* Discussion Paper. National Academy of Medicine.

Murali, N. & Sivakumaran, N. (2018) Artificial intelligence in healthcare – a review. *International Journal of Modern Computation, Information and Communication Technology*, 1(6), 103-110.

Nabi, J. (2018) Artificial intelligence can augment global pathology initiatives. *Lancet*, 392, 2351-2352.

Neill, D.B. (2013) Using artificial intelligence to improve hospital inpatient care. *IEEE Intelligent Systems*, March/April, 92-95.

Noguerol, T.M. et al. (2019) Strengths, weaknesses, opportunities, and threats analysis of artificial intelligence and machine learning applications in radiology. *Journal of the American College of Radiology*, 16 (9PB), 1239-1247.

Nordling, L. (2019) Mind the gap: artificial intelligence has great potential to improve healthcare, but without careful implementation, only a privileged portion of society will benefit. Nature, 573, S103-S105.

Nuffield Council on Bioethics (2018) Bioethics briefing note: artificial Intelligence in healthcare and research.

Obermeyer, Z. et al. (2019) Dissecting racial bias in an algorithm used to manage the health of populations. *Science*, 366 (64640, 447-453.

O'Mara, A., et al. (2015) Using text mining for study identification in systematic reviews: a systematic review of current approaches. *Syst Rev* 4, 5.

Oracle Health Services (2017) *mHealth and the transformation of clinical trials: harnessing data, advanced analytics, and the internet of things to optimise digitised clinical trials.* Oracle White Paper, June.

Palanisamy, V. & Thirunavukarasu, R. (2019) Implications of big data analytics in developing healthcare frameworks – a review. *Journal of King Saud University – Computer and Information Sciences*, 31, 415-425

Phaneuf, A. (2021) *Use of AI in healthcare & medicine is booming – here's how the medical field is benefiting from AI in 2021 and beyond.* Science. Business Insider.

Probst, L., Pedersen, B. & Dakkak-Arnoux, L. (2017) Harnessing the economic benefits of artificial intelligence. Digital Transformation Monitor, European Commission.

Protti, D. (2015) *Missed connections: the adoption of information technology in Canadian healthcare.* Commentary No. 422. Toronto: C.D. Howe Institute.

Raghupathi, W. & Raghupathi, V. (2014) Big data analytics in healthcare: promise and potential. *Health Information Science and Systems*, 2:3

Raheem, E. (2018) Introduction. *Journal of Biomedical Analytics*, 1(1), pp. 51-53.

Renwick, M., Simpkin, V. & Mossialos, E. (2016) *Targeting innovation in antibiotic drug discovery and development: the need for a one health – one Europe – one world framework.* Copenhagen: World Health Organization.

Ristevski, B. & Chen, M. (2018) Big data analytics in medicine and healthcare. *Journal of Integrative Bioinformatics*, 20170030.

Robin, N., Klein, T. & Jutting, J. (2016) *Public-private partnerships for statistics: lessons learned, future steps, OECD Development Co-operation Working Paper 27.* Paris: Organisation for Economic Cooperation and Development.

Rosa, C. et al. (2016) Using e-technologies in clinical trials. *Contemporary Clinical Trials*, 45(00), pp. 41-55.

Sanchez-Serrano, I., Pfeiffer, T. & Chaguturu, R. (2018) Disruptive approaches to accelerate drug discovery and development. *Drug Discovery World*, pp. 39-52.

Shahbaz, M., Gao, C., Zhai, L. et al. (2019) Investigating the adoption of big data analytics in healthcare: the moderating role of resistance to change. *Journal of Big Data*, 6:6 https://doi.org/10.1186/s40537-019-0170-y

Shearer, E., Stirling, R. et al. (2020) *Government AI readiness index 2020*. Oxford Insights.

Stanford University (2016) *Artificial intelligence and life in 2030: one hundred year study on artificial intelligence*. Report of the 2015 Study Panel 2016.

Stevens, H. et al. (2017) *Vaccines: accelerating innovation and access*. Global Challenges Report. World Intellectual Property Organization (WIPO).

Tait, A.R. et al. (2015) Using digital multimedia to improve parents' and children's understanding of clinical trials. *Arch Dis Child*, 100, 589-593.

The Economist Intelligence Unit (2018) *The innovation imperative: the future of drug development, part 1 – research methods and findings*. The Economist Corporate Network.

Thakur, D. (2018) *Artificial intelligence – the policy challenge for low and middle income countries*. World Wide Web Foundation. ITU-T SG3 Workshop on AI, Geneva.

Tierney, M. C. (2019) Embracing AI: Why now is the time for medical imaging. *AI in Healthcare*, 2(1), 1-27.

Tirziu, A.G. (2018) *Coming to life: artificial intelligence in Africa*. Atlantic Council – Africa Center. Issue Brief.

Twilt, M. (2016) Precision medicine: the new era in medicine. *EBioMedicine*, 4, 24-25.

USAID Center for Innovation and Impact (2019) The artificial intelligence in global health report – defining a collective path forward.

Wahl, B., Cossy-Gantner A., Germann S, *et al.* Artificial intelligence (AI) and global health: how can AI contribute to health in resource-poor settings? *BMJ Glob Health* 2018;3:e000798. doi:10.1136/bmjgh-2018-000798

Waithira, N., Mutinda, B. & Cheah, P.Y. (2019) Data management and sharing policy: the step towards promoting data sharing. *BMC Medicine*, 17:80. https://doi.org/10.1186/s12916-019-1315-8

Weng, H., Chen, H. & Wang, M. (2018) Innovation in neglected tropical disease drug discovery and development. *Infectious Diseases of Poverty*, 7:67.

WHO (2016) *Vaccines*. Health topics 2016.

Wibmer, A. et al. (2015) Haralick texture analysis of prostate MRI: utility for differentiating non-cancerous prostate cancer and differentiating prostate cancers with different Gleason scores. Eur Radiol, 25, 2840.

Wright, B. (2020) *AI in Africa faces hurdles: these 5 countries are leading the way*. CIO.

Wu, Y. et al. (2015) Multiple fuzzy c-means clustering algorithm in medical diagnosis. Technol Health Care, 23(Suppl 2), S519-27.

Don't miss out!

Visit the website below and you can sign up to receive emails whenever Mbuso Mabuza publishes a new book. There's no charge and no obligation.

https://books2read.com/r/B-A-JPJL-LYKIC

BOOKS 2 READ

Connecting independent readers to independent writers.

Did you love *Artificial Intelligence In Drug Discovery And Development*? Then you should read *The Journey of Life Has a Gift of Purpose*[1] by Mbuso Mabuza!

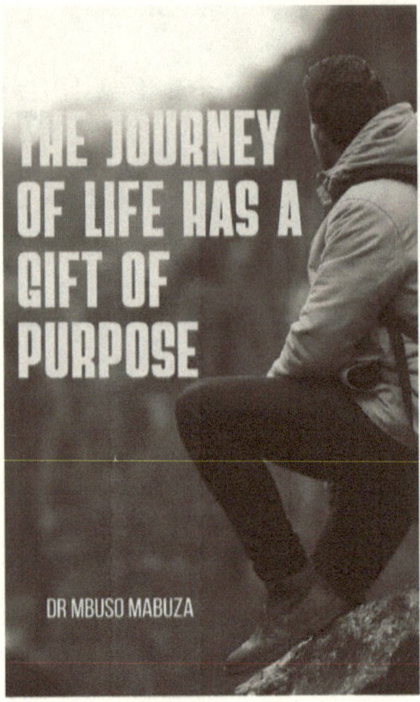

[2]

"Everything is guiding you to your authenticity. No matter what happens to you. It is all feedback and on the way. By asking quality questions that equilibrate the mind and liberate you from the bondage of pain, infatuation, resentment, and pride and shame, you are freed to be authentic, where you: love, feel inspired, are grateful, are present, are certain, and are enthused. In this state, you are capable of doing extraordinary feats." **Dr. John Demartini, Human Behaviour Expert**

Each day is a gift, and each day brings its own individual wonder. Understand the message in this gift and make the most of life.

---

1. https://books2read.com/u/mvXLnq

2. https://books2read.com/u/mvXLnq

Surely we ought to hold tightly to life, and also know when to let go, for it is wondrous, and full of a beauty that breaks through every pore of God's own earth. We know that this is so, but all too often we recognise this truth only in our backward glance when we remember what was and then suddenly realise it is no more.

To find meaning and significance in life, we must look back and observe the path we have taken. It will never be perfect, but we will surely find our own personal or professional achievements as well as those of others and society. It is the journey that is more important, and not the destination. Changing your attitude is crucial.

We can reflect on our journey away from the doom and gloom perspective, seeing instead an ocean of opportunity and prospects as self-actualised citizens. The capable and good in us must rise to the occasion. If we are to strive for true success, we must construct positive declarations written not only on paper, but on our hearts and conscious minds, inscribed in the animus of our existence as human beings, to act as rudders that will direct our paths. By doing so, we take control of setting into play what we desire to see as outcomes in our lives. The power and impact of our words wrought deep inside our core create unbreakable principles by which we can attain our highest values in life, business and society.

I challenge you to consider the infinite possibilities and to take control of your actions and the influences around you. Do not just go with the flow, but carve out a victorious path and inspire the same in others. Use your gifts and talents to serve with authenticity. Remember to prioritise your health and wellbeing as you journey along.

Sometimes, the journey of life may seem slow, painful, confusing, and energy-sapping, to such an extent that some people are all too ready to throw in the towel. Do not despair. Do not slack in your perseverance. Your mental shift can determine your destiny. If you want to change your life for the better, you need to stretch your mind. Value yourself, and face challenges with poise. Circumstances do not make you, but they reveal you.

What makes the value of anything in life? Not enjoyment, not possessions. Analyse everything. You will find that there is no value except – experience, to teach us something. And in many cases it is our hardships that give us better experience than enjoyment.

Your life is constantly under construction. There is always something to improve. You are here to make the world a better place. This life and its blessings has been given to us as a gift, to be passed on to others. To live your life in hatred is a lie. You came here to love. You came here to grow.

First of all, do no harm! The journey of life has a gift of purpose.

This book will be invaluable to every person who would like to live life to the fullest.

Also by Mbuso Mabuza

A Healthy Mind And Best You: Achieving Great Results in Every Aspect of Your Life
Purposeful And Better You
Efficacy, Effectiveness And Efficiency In The Management Of Health Systems
Promoting Health and Wellbeing
Medicine and the Sociology of Health
Qualitative Methods In Public Health Research
Global Health Disaster Management
Global Health Policy And Programme Challenges
The Journey of Life Has a Gift of Purpose
Epidemiological Research
Ethics, Qualitative And Quantitative Methods In Public Health Research
Emotional Intelligence in Relationships
Blockchain Technology In Healthcare And Medicine
Immersive Technologies In Healthcare: Virtual Reality And Augmented Reality
Health Data Analytics And Informatics
How To Improve The Way You Think
Health Systems Engineering
Artificial Intelligence In Drug Discovery And Development
How To Make The Most Of Life
Precision Medicine
Connected Health: Technology-Enabled Care

Person Centered Care And Optimal Wellbeing
Reimagine Your Tomorrow
Leading Remote Teams in the 21st Century
Qualitative Research In Health and Medicine
Excellence In Medicine

About the Author

Dr Mbuso Mabuza is a highly motivated life-long learner and multi-skilled global health professional. Dr Mabuza's mission is to improve health outcomes and to expand quality healthcare experiences amongst all groups of people and influence change and innovation.

www.ingramcontent.com/pod-product-compliance
Lightning Source LLC
LaVergne TN
LVHW090430210926
848480LV00002B/759